Vegan Diet

Vegan Diet And Recipes For Ultimate Weight Loss

Michelle Goodfield

© 2016

Table of Contents

© Copyright 2016 by Michelle Goodfield - All rights reserved.

This document is geared towards providing exact and reliable information in regards to the topic and issue covered. The publication is sold with the idea that the publisher is not required to render accounting, officially permitted, or otherwise, qualified services. If advice is necessary, legal or professional, a practiced individual in the profession should be ordered.

- From a Declaration of Principles which was accepted and approved equally by a Committee of the American Bar Association and a Committee of Publishers and Associations.

In no way is it legal to reproduce, duplicate, or transmit any part of this document in either electronic means or in printed format. Recording of this publication is strictly prohibited and any storage of this document is not allowed unless with written permission from the publisher. All rights reserved.

The information provided herein is stated to be truthful and consistent, in that any liability, in terms of inattention or otherwise, by any usage or abuse of any policies, processes, or directions contained within is the solitary and utter responsibility of the recipient reader. Under no circumstances will any legal responsibility or blame be held against the publisher for any reparation, damages, or monetary loss due to the information herein, either directly or indirectly.

Respective authors own all copyrights not held by the publisher.

The information herein is offered for informational purposes solely, and is universal as so. The presentation of the information is without contract or any type of guarantee assurance.

The trademarks that are used are without any consent, and the publication of the trademark is without permission or backing by the trademark owner. All trademarks and brands within this book are for clarifying purposes only and are the owned by the owners themselves, not affiliated with this document.

Introduction

Going on a diet can be tough. You need to figure out the foods that you are allowed to eat and which ones you will need to avoid to see success on the diet. You may also need to consider some different cooking methods, whether this diet is supposed to work with the specific needs you are looking for, and whether you will be able to keep up with all of the work that comes with it.

The Vegan diet is a great option for you to choose when you are looking for a diet plan that will fit your needs. It is full of fantastic fruits and vegetable options along with some of the tastiest meals that you could look for in a diet plan. With all the healthy foods that you will start to eat when you go on this diet plan, you will be able to cure many of the illnesses that plague most of the country today. Plus you are going to be able to lose weight and feel great once you get used to this diet plan.

Of course, you will need to give up some of your favorite foods along the way to ensure that you are following the Vegan diet, and this can sometimes be the hardest part. Meat products and their byproducts are a part of the American culture and thinking about getting rid of them for the long term can be hard, which is sometimes why people fail, or at least slowly ease into the process. But with some practice, and some great recipes, this is a diet plan that you are going to love for the great tastes as well as the great results.

This guidebook is going to take some time to go through the Vegan diet by discussing what this diet entails as well as some of the benefits of going with this diet instead of another one. We will then explore some of the best recipes that you can enjoy while on this diet, including options for breakfast, lunch, and dinner so you feel full and satisfied rather than worried about when your next meal is.

While the Vegan diet may be a tough one to get used to, once you do a little research about all the benefits and learn some of the best recipes that you can enjoy while on this diet, it becomes much easier than you would expect. Use this guidebook to get started on the Vegan diet and learn just how great this diet can work, as well as how great some of the recipes will taste while you are getting healthy.

Chapter 1: What is the Vegan Diet?

The Vegan diet is probably one of the most misunderstood diets in the world. Many people have no idea what all this diet entails and they are going to miss out on a wonderfully healthy way of living, rather than just a diet that helps them lose weight before adding it all back on again. The vegan diet is basically a form of abstinence from using animal products both in your lifestyle and in your diet.

Veganism is a way of life that is going to exclude, at least as much as possible, any forms of cruelty and exploitation for animals either for clothing, food, or other purposes. While some people choose to go all out and won't use cosmetics, hair products, or clothes that were made from animals, many people will focus more on the diet part where they will not eat foods that come from animas including honey, animal milks, eggs, poultry, fish, and meat.

Why Choose Veganism?

The first question that many vegans are asked is why choose this lifestyle. Isn't it a hard one to maintain while trying to find good foods to eat or picking out the clothes and other products that you would like to use on a regular basis? While it may pose a bit of a challenge, there are many great reasons why you may choose to adopt the vegan lifestyle including:

- Objecting to animals being used as commodities and being concerned about the welfare of animals
- Environmental issues. These could include that the factories using the animals are contaminating the water or polluting the air.
- Ending world hunger. With veganism, the person is learning how to efficiently use the food resources within the planet rather than wasting what we have left.

What to Eat

So, while you are on the Vegan diet, you will need to get rid of the animal products that you are consuming in order to do it properly. To many people, this may seem like a big limitation to what they are allowed to eat, but with some practice and thinking things through, you will find there are still plenty of things that you can enjoy. Some of the foods that you can enjoy while on the vegan diet include:

- All types of fruits. This could include options like papaya, grapes, pineapple, mangoes, berries, oranges, and apples
- All types of vegetables including spinach, zucchini, celery, carrots, broccoli, kale, and asparagus.
- Nuts and seeds of all kinds including the butter made from them.
- Carbohydrates that are found within quinoa, rice, wraps, pitas, bagels, breads, pasta, and potatoes.
- Beans and legumes

- Non-dairy milks such as oat milk, soy milk, almond milk, and coconut milk.
- Chocolate that is made out of dark chocolate as well as any variety that is made from non-dairy sources.
- Dairy alternatives such as almond yogurt, coffee creamers, vegan butter, and coconut ice cream are just some examples.
- Meat alternatives including holiday roasts, vegan sausages, veggie burgers and so on.

Since more and more people are becoming fans of the vegan diet, more products are becoming available to help fit this lifestyle. This makes it easier for consumers to find the products that they want while still maintaining their new lifestyle.

What Should I Avoid?

The Vegan diet is a bit more restrictive than other diets, but it is to help you keep the environment safe and secure. Some of the things that you are going to need to avoid if you wish to follow the vegan lifestyle include:

- Any products that have been tested on animals
- Fabrics that have been derived from animals including wool and silk
- Any animal product, such as beef, chicken, or fish, as well as their byproducts such as honey or milk.
- Fur, down, suede, and leather
- Any personal care products that will have an animal ingredient including keratin, beeswax, and lanolin.

- Animals that are used in entertainment including rodeos and circuses.

As you can see, following all of this completely is really hard for most people to do. For example, most clothes are made out of at least a bit of cotton so finding something to wear could be impossible if you went on this kind of diet. This is why most people don't follow a completely vegan lifestyle, but will focus more on the diet part, such as cutting out all of the meat products and byproducts from their menus, and then do what they can to avoid the other things listed above.

Chapter 2: The Health And Weight Loss Benefits Of The Vegan Diet

While the Vegan diet may seem like one that is hard to follow, there are so many great benefits that can come from this diet choice. Going with a plant and fruit based diet can give you so many great nutrients and antioxidants that it is hard to see why you didn't go on the diet before. Let's explore some of the great health benefits that you will get when you choose to go on the Vegan diet.

Health Benefits of Veganism

There are a lot of great benefits that can come from choosing to go on this kind of diet. Some of the great benefits include:

- Reduce risk of disease—studies have shown that there are fewer chronic diseases in those who choose to follow a vegan diet compared to those in other groups.
- Less likely to get diabetes—since you aren't eating a lot of processed foods and other foods that can raise your blood sugars, you are less likely to get diabetes.
- Keeps body weight healthy—you are cutting out a lot of the bad foods that you may have enjoyed before, such as fast food, and replacing with fruits and vegetables, making it easier to keep your body at a healthy weight.
- Lower heart disease—many meat options, such as beef, can add cholesterol and bad fats to

your body. When you reduce these and replace with produce, you are keeping the heart strong.

- Reduce the risk of cancer—the higher intake of antioxidants in the produce you are eating can help to keep away the cancer cells. This is especially true when it comes to cancer in the digestive tract.
- Helps the thyroid—veganism seems to help protect the individual from hypothyroidism. While you may have to combine in with some other health changes, it can help you to keep health.
- Reduce the risk of cataracts—the vegan diet is great at helping to keep your eyesight right where it should be. This could be because of all the healthy nutrients you are getting in.
- Helps with rheumatoid arthritis—a study done in 2010 suggests that the vegan diet is able to help improve the symptoms that come with rheumatoid arthritis. This could be due to the nutrients you are now getting in that help to keep the inflammation away.
- Healthy kidneys—the vegan diet is able to help balance the phosphate levels in your body and will keep the acidity levels low. These help the kidneys remain healthy.
- Extends your life—the high amount of nutrients that are available in a vegan diet can help you to live longer since your metabolic health is higher than many others.

Veganism and Weight Loss

Chances are you are looking at this diet in order to lose some weight. Whether you just want to lose a few pounds and be healthier or you are more interested in getting a lot of weight off, the Vegan diet may be the best choice for you.

It is possible to lose some weight on the Vegan diet; the amount that you lose will depend on how closely you stick with the diet as well as what other factors, such as exercise, you start to introduce into your life. You are going to start adding in a lot of healthy fruits and vegetables, while getting rid of other options, such as meat and their byproducts which can be really unhealthy for you. You will no longer be eating out and all those antioxidants that you will consume can help you to feel your best in no time.

Keep in mind that with the weight loss, you should expect to average between one and two pounds a week. This is a safe amount to ensure that you are steadily able to lose the weight without gaining it all back. While you may lose a little more in the beginning since you are switching off all that bad food and detoxing the body, it will average out to be a bit steadier in the long run.

You will also need to start with an exercise program. If you have a lot of weight to lose and haven't been on an exercise program in the past, start out small. Walking a few times a day can make a big difference as can doing some basic yoga or some light weights. Over time you can increase the duration and the intensity, but anything is better than nothing and will aid in the weight loss.

When you want to lose weight or get some of your other health problems in line and other diets are not working for you, this may be the one that you should try out. You are feeding your body a lot of fantastic and whole foods that you aren't able to get in some other diets and with all the nutrients out of the produce, this could be the way to lose weight quickly and get your health back on track the way that you would like.

While using this diet plan, make sure that you follow it in a healthy way. Going with canned fruit, while technically vegan, is not that healthy with all the extra sugars that are inside and you won't see as many of the results as you would like. In addition, you should take some time to begin an exercise program in here to really tone the muscles and to ensure that you are losing the weight in a natural way. If you are unsure about the types of food that you should be eating or about what kinds of exercises work the best for your body during this time, consider finding someone who had done this diet and can help you out.

Not only are you going to see some great results when it comes to your weight loss on this diet program, but you will get the chance to see some amazing health benefits as well. Those who have gone on this diet and been successful have had the chance to reverse their issues with diabetes, limit the pain from arthritis and other inflammation issues, and even to help keep their heart strong. Who knew that eating fruit in this manner and getting rid of many of the bad foods that you typically enjoy in your diet could be so great for every part of your body.

You should remember that the Vegan diet is a tough one to follow. You are giving up several food groups to maintain this diet and it is hard for some people. Perhaps consider going Vegan for one or two days a week to get used to the idea and slowly switch over. This makes it easier and you won't feel so deprived in the long run.

Chapter 3: Vegan Breakfasts To Burn Belly Fat

Kale Frittata

Ingredients:

Pepper
Salt
¼ c. almond milk
4 Tbsp. nutritional yeast
1 Tbsp. Dijon mustard
4 Tbsp. cornstarch
5 oz. silken tofu
5 oz. crumbled firm tofu
6 kale leaves, chopped
4 chopped green onions
1 chopped garlic clove
1 chopped shallot
4 Tbsp. olive oil

Directions:

1. Heat up some oil in a skillet and stir the garlic and shallot inside. Cook for about 2 minutes to make translucent and soft.
2. Add in the crumbled tofu and allow it to turn brown.
3. Take out a blender and pulse together the silken tofu with the almond milk, mustard, and nutritional yeast. Mix in the kale and the green onions and season a bit before adding into the skillet.

4. Turn the heat to a low setting and cook for 10 minutes on one side. Flip the frittata over and continue cooking for another 10 minutes before serving.

Raisin Pudding

Ingredients:

Salt
4 Tbsp. agave syrup
1 tsp. vanilla
½ c. golden raisins
1 tsp. cinnamon
1 c. apple juice
2 c. water
1 c. quinoa

Directions:

1. Take out a pan and pour the apple juice and water inside, bringing to boil. Add in the raisins and the quinoa and cook so the liquid becomes absorbed.
2. At this time, take the pot from the heat and add in the agave, salt, cinnamon, and vanilla. Allow it to cool down a bit before serving.

Pumpkin French Toast

Ingredients:

¼ c. coconut oil
¼ tsp. cinnamon powder
¼ c. almond milk
1 c. pumpkin puree

4 slices sandwich bread

Directions:

1. Combine together the cinnamon, almond milk, and pumpkin puree.
2. Place each slice of bread into the mixture, making sure to get all sides soaked.
3. Heat up the oil in a pan and drop down each slice. Cook for a few minutes to make the one side golden brown before flipping and doing the same on the other side.
4. Drain off the excess oil and serve with some syrup or other topping of choice.

Peanut Butter Banana Bars

Ingredients:

½ c. chopped cranberries
1 pinch ginger
1 pinch nutmeg
½ tsp. cinnamon powder
¼ c. flour, whole wheat
3 c. rolled oats
2 Tbsp. ground flax seeds
4 Tbsp. agave syrup
½ c. almond milk
½ c. peanut butter
2 mashed bananas

Directions:

1. Mix together the flax seeds, syrup, milk, peanut butter, and bananas to combine. When ready,

add in the salt, ginger, nutmeg, cinnamon, flour, and oats.
2. When this is well combined, fold the cranberries in and spoon the whole thing into a square pan.
3. Turn the oven on to 350 degrees and bake the bars for 30 minutes. Allow them to cool down in the pan once done and then slice into squares before serving.

Blueberry and Banana Bread

Ingredients:

½ c. almond milk
½ c. agave syrup
1 Tbsp. lemon juice
3 mashed bananas
½ tsp. cinnamon
½ tsp. baking soda
1 tsp. baking powder
1 pinch salt
½ c. almond meal
2 c. flour
1 c. blueberries
1 tsp. vanilla

Directions:

1. Inside a bowl, mix together the cinnamon, baking soda, baking powder, salt, almond meal, and flour.
2. Inside another bowl, combine the vanilla, almond milk, agave syrup, lemon juice, and bananas.

3. Pour the liquids on top of the other bowl and mix together well. Turn the oven on to 350 while you pour the batter into an oven proof pan.
4. Cook the bread for 40 minutes before taking out of the oven and allowing to cool.
5. Transfer to a rack and then slice before serving.

Cranberry Scones

Ingredients:

1 c. chopped cranberries
2/3 c. coconut oil
1 c. applesauce
2 Tbsp. sugar
¼ tsp. ginger
1 pinch nutmeg
1 pinch salt
1 tsp. baking soda
1 tsp. baking powder
½ c. almond meal
1 c. all purpose flour
1 c. whole wheat flour

Directions:

1. Mix together the sugar, ground ginger, nutmeg, salt, baking soda and powder, almond meal and the flours. Stir in the coconut oil and then rub together until the mixture is crumbly.
2. Slowly pour in the applesauce and mix so it becomes like a dough. Add in the cranberries and then knead the dough.
3. Move this to a working surface and shape into a sheet. Using a knife, you can cut the dough into

triangles and then arrange onto a prepared baking sheet.
4. Turn on the oven to 375 degrees and bake the scones for 20 minutes or until done. Serve with some jam and enjoy!

Breakfast Time Waffles

Ingredients:

Salt
4 Tbsp. coconut oil
1 pinch nutmeg
1 tsp. cinnamon powder
1 tsp. vanilla
2 bananas
2 c. almond milk
½ c. ground walnuts
2 c. oatmeal

1. Combine together all of your ingredients inside a blender until they are smooth.
2. Prepare the waffle maker and then add in some of the batter to the hot machine.
3. Cook the waffles until well done and then take out to cool down. Repeat the steps with the rest of the batter.
4. Serve these with fresh fruit or other toppings that you like.

Chapter 4: Vegan Loveable Lunches To Keep You Full And Happy

Avocado Burgers

Ingredients:

1 lettuce leaf
1 sliced tomato
4 burger buns
1 avocado, sliced
Pepper
Salt
½ c. breadcrumbs
1 tsp. thyme
2 chopped green onions
¼ tsp. chili flakes
4 garlic cloves
2 c. black beans
2 c. lentils, canned

Directions:

1. Combine together the thyme, green onions, chili flakes, and garlic in a blender for 2 minutes to combine well.
2. Move this over to a bowl and stir in the breadcrumbs and the lentils. Add a bit more pepper and salt to get the taste that you are looking for.
3. Form the burgers into the size that you want and place them onto a prepared baking pan.

Turn the oven on to 400 degrees and bake the burgers for 15 minutes.

4. When this is done, serve on the hamburger buns with a tomato, lettuce leaf, and avocado slice and enjoy.

Mediterranean Gazpacho

Ingredients:

Pepper
Salt
1 tsp. oregano
1 tsp. basil
2 Tbsp. coriander, chopped
¼ c. chopped parsley
1 tsp. agave syrup
1 tsp. apple cider vinegar
1 sliced red bell pepper
1 celery stalk
2 garlic cloves
1 shallot
½ cucumber
4 tomatoes, seeded

Directions:

1. Bring out your blender and place the agave syrup, vinegar, bell pepper, celery, garlic, shallot, cucumber, and tomatoes inside. Process these for a few minutes to make them smooth.
2. Fold in the rest of the ingredients before pouring into the serving bowls. Serve this right away.

Tofu Spring Rolls

Ingredients

Rolls
1 bunch cilantro
1 sliced zucchini
1 sliced celery stalk
2 sliced carrots
10 oz. sliced tofu
16 soaked rice wrappers
Sauce
Pepper
Salt
1 drop chili sauce
½ tsp. garlic powder
1 tsp. ginger, grated
2 Tbsp. lemon juice
¼ c. peanut butter

Directions:

1. Start out by making the rolls. Take each of the wrappers and place some of the vegetables into each one. Bring two of the edges to the middle and wrap them up.
2. Heat up some oil and fry the rolls to make them crisp and golden.
3. To make the sauce, combine all of your ingredients into a bowl and mix well, adding in more pepper and salt if needed.
4. Arrange your prepared rolls on a platter and add the dip to the middle before serving.

Quinoa and Fennel Salad

Ingredients:

Pepper
Salt
¼ c. coriander, chopped
½ c. orange segments
4 Tbsp. olive oil
2 Tbsp. lemon juice
1 fennel bulb, sliced
3 c. vegetable stock
1 c. quinoa

Directions:

1. Put the vegetable stock into a pan and let it come to boil. Add in the quinoa and cook until it is done. Give it some time to cool down.
2. Heat up a few tablespoons of olive oil on a skillet and add the fennel. Cook this for about 10 minutes to make the fennel tender before taking off the heat.
3. To finish your salad, combine the quinoa with the coriander, fennel, and orange segments and then gently mix before serving.

Cauliflower and Rice Pilaf

Ingredients:

¼ c. coriander, chopped
1 bay leaf
1 cinnamon stick
4 c. vegetable stock
1 c. basmati rice
1 head cauliflower, cut up
½ tsp. cumin powder

½ tsp. turmeric powder
1 tsp. curry powder
2 chopped garlic cloves
1 chopped shallot
2 Tbsp. coconut oil

Directions:

1. Heat up some coconut oil in a skillet and add in the garlic and shallot. Cook these until they are soft and then add in the turmeric, cumin, curry powder, cinnamon stick, and bay leaf.
2. Cook these ingredients for another minute before adding the rice and cauliflower and pouring in the stock.
3. Cover up the pan and cook everything for about 30 minutes or until the rice is done.
4. When it is done, add in the coriander and then serve this right away or chill until later.

Caesar Salad

Ingredients:

2 toasted and cubed bread slices
Pepper
Salt
2 garlic cloves
½ lemon juiced
½ c. cashew nuts, soaked
4 Tbsp. olive oil
6 oz. sliced tofu, firm
1 lettuce head, shredded

Directions:

1. Heat up a grill pan and brush on a bit of olive oil. Add in the slices of tofu and cook so both sides can become browned. Take out of the pan and set to the side.
2. Work on the sauce next. To do this, mix together the rest of the olive oil, garlic, lemon juice, and cashew nuts in a blender. Process this for a few minutes so that your sauce becomes creamy and thick. Add in a bit more lemon juice to intensify the flavor.
3. Arrange the lettuce onto a plate and top with the tofu slices and drizzle with some of the sauce. Add on some bread cubes and serve right away.

Sweet Potato Curry

Ingredients:

Pepper
Salt
2 c. shredded spinach leaves
1 c. vegetable stock
1 c. coconut milk
2 sliced carrots
2 c. cauliflower
3 cubed sweet potatoes
2 tsp. curry paste
1 tsp. ginger
2 chopped garlic cloves
1 sliced onion
4 Tbsp. olive oil

Directions:

1. Heat up some oil in a skillet before adding in the garlic and onion and cooking for about two minutes to make soft. Add in the curry paste and ginger and cook for another minute.
2. At this time, add in the vegetables as well as the stock and the coconut milk. Put the lid on the pot and cook for about 40 minutes so the sauce is reduced a bit and the vegetables are soft.
3. Right before taking the pot off the heat, add in the spinach and then serve warm.

Chapter 5: Vegan Dinners To Aid Weight Loss

Italian Pasta

Ingredients:

Pepper
Salt
2 garlic cloves
1 Tbsp. lemon juice
¼ c. olive oil
¼ c. walnuts
¼ c. pine nuts
1 c. basil leaves
15 oz. spaghetti

Directions:

1. Inside your blender, combine the pepper, salt, garlic, lemon juice, walnuts, pine nuts, and basil until smooth, slowly adding in the olive oil as you go. Set this to the side.
2. Pour some water into a pot and bring it to a boil. Cook the spaghetti by following the instructions on the bag. Drain out the water when done and move over to a bowl.
3. Pour the pesto on top of the pasta and toss around to coat. Serve right away.

Tofu Steak

Ingredients:

4 Tbsp. olive oil
1.4 c. parsley, chopped
2 Tbsp. balsamic vinegar
2 minced garlic cloves
4 Portobello mushrooms
2 Tbsp. olive oil
1 Tbsp. lemon juice
1 Tbsp. soy sauce
4 firm slices tofu

Directions:

1. Take out a bowl and mix together the 2 tablespoons of olive oil, lemon juice, and soy sauce. Brush this onto the tofu slices.
2. Prepare a grill pan before adding in the tofu and grilling on both sides for about 4 minutes.
3. In that pan, place the mushrooms and cook to make tender. Move the mushrooms over to a bowl and mix together with the leftover olive oil, garlic, parsley, and balsamic vinegar. Mix to coat the mushrooms.
4. Serve the tofu steak with the mushrooms and enjoy.

Ratatouille

Ingredients:

¼ c. olive oil
2 c. diced tomatoes, canned
1 tsp. thyme
1 tsp. cumin powder
1 c. drained black beans
1 c. drained chickpeas, canned
1 sliced onion

2 cubed sweet potatoes
2 sliced bell peppers
1 cubed eggplant
2 sliced zucchinis

Directions:

1. Layer the vegetables into a baking dish and sprinkle with some salt, thyme, cumin, and pepper, drizzling with olive oil.
2. Turn the oven to 350 degrees and when it is hot, bake the vegetables for an hour.
3. Serve this warm with some garnish if you prefer and enjoy.

Vegan Pot Pie

Ingredients:

Filling
2 Tbsp. cornstarch
1 diced potato
2 chopped garlic cloves
3 c. green peas
1 diced carrot
1 chopped shallot
6 oz. diced tofu
2 Tbsp. olive oil
1 ½ c. vegetable stock
Crust
½ c. coconut oil
½ c. applesauce
1 pinch baking powder
1 pinch salt
2 ½ c. flour

Directions:

1. Work on the crusts first. To do this, combine the baking powder and salt in the bowl before adding the coconut oil and stirring until crumbly.
2. Add in the apple sauce and stir so you get a kind of dough and then shape into a ball. Wrap up in plastic until you are ready to use it.
3. To work on the filling, heat some oil inside a skillet and stir in the garlic and shallot for 2 minutes. Add in the green peas, potato, carrot, and tofu and cook for an additional ten minutes.
4. Mix the vegetable stock with your cornstarch and pour on top of the veggies, continuing to cook so it thickens.
5. Spoon your filling into 6 ramekins and set to the side.
6. Take out the crust and roll it out onto a working surface until thin. Cut into small rounds and place on top of the vegetables.
7. Turn the oven on to 375 degrees and bake the pot pies for about 30 minutes or until they are done. Serve these warm and enjoy!

Tempeh Fajitas

Ingredients:

2 chopped garlic cloves
1 chopped shallot
½ sliced chili pepper
2 c. spinach leaves
2 s. sliced mushrooms
1 sliced bell pepper yellow

1 sliced bell pepper, red
1 Tbsp. soy sauce
10 oz. cubed tempeh
2 Tbsp. olive oil

Directions:

1. Heat up the oil inside a skillet and add in the garlic and shallot. Cook these ingredients for 2 minute until soft and then add in the rest of the ingredients.
2. Cook this on a low heat for about 20 minutes so the liquids are reduced and your vegetables become tender.
3. Serve these warm, adding in a few more spices if you would like.

Vegan Goulash

Ingredients:

½ c. tomato puree
2 c. vegetable stock
¼ c. red wine
1 lb. cubed potatoes
5 oz. green beans
1 bay leaf
½ tsp. cumin powder
1 ½ tsp. paprika
2 chopped garlic cloves
5 oz. cubed tofu
2 sliced bell peppers, red
1 chopped onion, red
2 Tbsp. olive oil

Directions:

1. Heat up the olive oil in a skillet or big pot and stir in the garlic and the onion. Cook these so they become translucent and soft before adding in the tofu and the bell peppers.
2. Cook all of this for another five minutes before adding in the cumin powder, paprika, tomato puree, vegetable stock, red wine, potatoes, and green beans.
3. Now you can add in the pepper, salt, and bay leaf and turn the heat down to low. Cook for another hour or until the ingredients are soft. Serve this warm and enjoy!

Zucchini Lasagna

Ingredients

4 tomatoes, diced
½ c. chopped basil
2 Tbsp. lemon juice
1 tsp. garlic powder
½ c. soymilk
4 Tbsp. nutritional yeast
2 c. silken tofu
4 c. steamed spinach
3 sliced zucchinis

Directions:

1. Take out the blender and combine the tofu with the lemon juice, garlic powder, soymilk, and nutritional yeast. Combine this to make it creamy and smooth.
2. Inside a bowl, combine the pepper, salt, basil, and tomatoes together and set to the side.

3. Bring out a baking pan and place a few zucchini slices on the bottom. Top with some of the diced tomatoes and then add some sauce on top. Continue layering in this way until all the ingredients are gone.
4. Turn on the oven to 350 degrees and bake the lasagna until the vegetables are tender and ready. Take the pan form the oven and give it a few minutes to cool down before slicing and serving.

Tempeh Meatballs

Ingredients:

Tempeh Balls
1 c. breadcrumbs
1 tsp. basil
1 tsp. oregano
1 tsp. ginger
1 Tbsp. Dijon mustard
1 tsp. soy sauce
1 c. water
10 oz. tempeh
Tomato Sauce
2 Tbsp. olive oil
½ sliced chili pepper
1 c. vegetable stock
2 c. tomato puree
Pepper
1 tsp. capers
2 garlic cloves
1 chopped shallot

Directions:

1. Start by making the tempeh balls. Combine your tempeh with the pepper, salt, basil, oregano, ginger, mustard, soy sauce, and water. Place into a blender and pulse to blend before adding in the breadcrumbs.
2. After wetting your hands, form the tempeh into small balls and place them onto a baking tray before setting aside.
3. Make the sauce by heating up the olive oil in a skillet and stir in the garlic and shallot. Cook these for two minutes before adding in the stock and tomato puree. Add in the capers and the chili pepper and cook for another ten minutes.
4. At this time, add in the tempeh balls and lower the heat. Cook for 15 minutes, adding in a bit more stock if needed for the sauce.
5. Serve this as it is or add some mashed potatoes and enjoy!

Stuffed Zucchini and Eggplant

Ingredients:

10 zucchini
1 tsp. salt
1 tsp. rice spice
½ c. olive oil
1 onion
3 tomatoes
3 c. white rice
10 eggplants

Directions:

1. Place rice inside a bowl and let it soak for an hour. During this time, scoop out most of the flesh from the zucchini and the eggplants and then wash them out before laying onto a tray.
2. When the rice is ready, drain it and wash again before draining. Chop the onions into smaller cubes and add into the rice along with the tomatoes, salt, spices, and olive oil.
3. Stuff this into the eggplants and the zucchini and place into the pot, pouring the crushed tomatoes on top and adding a bit of salt. Add in some water to about half an inch above your vegetables.
4. Cook this on a high heat to get to boiling before reducing a bit and cooking for another 45 minutes. Serve right away.

Chapter 6: Vegan Delectable Desserts Low In Calories

Banana Fritters

Ingredients:
Fritters
1 ½ c. coconut oil
1 tsp. vanilla
1 pinch salt
½ c. almond milk
1 Tbsp. flax seeds
¼ tsp. baking powder
1 c. flour
4 sliced bananas
Caramel Sauce
2 Tbsp. coconut oil
1 c. coconut sugar
1 c. coconut milk
Salt

Directions:

1. Start by making the fritters. Combine together the salt, baking powder, flax seeds, and flour. Add in the vanilla and the almond milk and mix well.
2. Heat up some coconut oil in a pot. Dip the bananas into your prepared batter and drop them into the hot oil. Cook for a few minutes to make golden brown and then set aside.
3. Make the sauce next. Melt the coconut sugar in a pan and then add in the milk and coconut oil

and salt. Keep this on heat so it caramelized and melts. Allow to cool a bit.
4. To serve, place some of the fritters into a bowl and then drizzle on the caramel. Enjoy warm!

Vegan Chocolate Chip Cookies

Ingredients:

1 c. chocolate chips, vegan
1 tsp. vanilla
¼ c. almond milk
2/3 c. coconut oil
¼ c. peanut butter
1 c. raw sugar
2 tsp. baking powder
4 Tbsp. ground flax seeds
1 pinch salt
2 c. flour

Directions:

1. In a bowl, combine the sugar, baking powder, flax seeds, and salt. In another bowl, combine the peanut butter, vanilla, almond milk, and coconut oil and heat up in the microwave for a few seconds.
2. Pour the wet ingredients into the dry ones and then mix well to combine. Slowly fold in your chocolate chips.
3. Prepare some baking trays and then drop small amounts of the batter into the pan, leaving a bit of room for the cookies to spread.
4. Turn on the oven to 350 degrees and bake the cookies for about 15 minutes so they become

crisp. Allow these to cool down for a bit before serving.

Chocolate Pudding

Ingredients:

1 pinch salt
¼ c. coconut, shredded
¼ c. coconut milk
4 Tbsp. agave syrup
3 Tbsp. cocoa powder, raw
15 oz. silken tofu

Directions:

1. Combine the tofu with your other ingredients inside the blender and then process them together until the mixture is smooth.
2. Spoon this into your serving cups and place into the fridge to chill for an hour.
3. Add some coconut flakes on top before serving.

Cinnamon Rolls

Ingredients:

Dough
1 c. maple syrup
1 tsp. vanilla
1 ½ c. pumpkin puree, canned
1 Tbsp. apple cider vinegar
2 c. almond milk
½ c. coconut oil
Salt
3 tsp. active dry yeast

6 c. flour
Filling
1 c. peanut butter
½ c. maple syrup
2 tsp. cinnamon powder

Directions:

1. Work on the dough first. To do this, mix the yeast and the warm milk and let this set for 10 minutes. Stir in the maple syrup, pumpkin puree, vanilla, vinegar, and coconut oil.
2. Slowly add in the flour and some salt and knead the dough for ten minutes or so to get it elastic and easier to work with.
3. Cover the dough and let it rise for an hour so it starts to double.
4. While that is being done, work on the filling. Mix the maple syrup with the cinnamon and peanut butter.
5. When the dough is ready, roll it out into a thin sheet and spread the filling all around. Roll up the dough and then cut into slices before placing onto a prepared baking dish.
6. Allow the dough to rise for another 15 minutes while the oven heats up to 375 degrees.
7. Place the rolls into the oven and bake for about 20 minutes. Give the rolls some time to cool down before serving.

Chocolate Cupcakes

Ingredients:

Cupcakes
Salt

1 Tbsp. vanilla
½ c. hot water
½ c. coconut oil
½ tsp. baking soda
1 tsp. baking powder
½ c. cocoa powder
2/3 c. raw sugar
2/3 c. flour
1 c. rice flour
¼ c. water
2 Tbsp. ground flax seeds
Frosting
1 c. coconut, shredded
¼ c. coconut milk
3 c. sugar
½ c. coconut oil

Directions:

1. Work on the cupcakes first by mixing together the water and flax seeds in a bowl and letting them soak for 5 minutes.
2. Inside another bowl, combine the salt, baking soda and powder, cocoa powder, sugar, all purpose flour, and rice powder. Add in the rest of the ingredients as well and mix so the batter becomes smooth.
3. Pour this into a prepared muffin pan, leaving a bit of room at the beginning. Turn the oven on to 350 degrees and bake the cupcakes for about 15 minutes.
4. Work on the frosting next. Mix the coconut oil with the sugar so it becomes fluffy and white. Add in the sugar slowly before adding in the coconut milk.

5. Take one of your cupcakes when it is cool and cover with a bit of frosting. Roll in some shredded coconut and place out on a platter. Do these steps with the rest of the cupcakes and serve when ready.

Tofu Cheesecake

Ingredients

Crust
1 c. coconut
1 pinch salt
½ c. pitted dates
1 c. pecans
Filling
Salt
1 Tbsp. vanilla
2 Tbsp. cornstarch
½ c. agave syrup
10 oz. silken tofu
2 Tbsp. lemon juice
1 ½ c. cashew nuts, soaked over night
Topping
2 c. berries, fresh

Directions:

1. Start on the crust. To do this, combine the dates, slat, coconut, and pecans and pulse to make into a dough. Bring out a cake pan and press this into the bottom using your fingertips. Set this aside.
2. Work on the filling next. Place the soaked cashew nuts in a blender and add in the lemon juice. Combine until smooth before adding in

the salt, vanilla, cornstarch, agave syrup, and silken tofu. Pulse so it becomes smooth and then pour into the crust.

3. Turn the oven on to 350 degrees and then bake the cheesecake for about 40 minutes or until it set in the middle.
4. When the cheesecake is done, let it cool down before moving to a platter and topping with the fresh fruit. Slice it up and then serve.

Apple and Carrot Cake

Ingredients:

1 ½ c. water
1 bag baking powder
1 c. spelt flour
1 c. whole flour
1 Tbsp. cinnamon
2 bananas
1 c. brown sugar
¾ c. oil
3 carrots
3 apples

Directions:

1. Cut up one of the apples and the bananas and place into the blender along with a cup of water. Blend to make liquid.
2. Grate up your carrots until they are fine and place into a bowl. Cut up the other two apples with their pealing so they are in small cubes and then add into the carrots.

3. Place this mixture into the blender as well adding another ½ cup of water and the sugar and oil. Mix for two minutes.
4. In another bowl, add the baking powder, both flours, and the cinnamon. Add this to a mixer bowl slowly so you get an even texture. Add the apple and carrots to the mixture along with the banana and apple and continue to mix to get combined.
5. Prepare a baking pan and pour the batter inside. Turn on the oven to 350 degrees and bake the cake for about 35 minutes or until it is done. Serve warm or store for later.

Conclusion

The Vegan diet is probably one of the most misunderstood diets available right now. Many people just don't understand how this diet plan is supposed to work or they will assume that the diet is just too hard for them to handle. While this is not the easiest diet for you to choose, if you are looking for a great way to get your health in check while taking care of the environment at the same time, there is nothing better than the Vegan diet.

One of the biggest issues with going on a diet like the Vegan diet is finding the right recipes that will help you get started and see some results. This guidebook is going to take all the guesswork out of that by providing you with some of the best recipes that you are going to love that also follow the Vegan diet. You are not going to feel deprived or like you are missing out on flavor when you choose one of these dishes and you will soon wonder why you didn't go on the Vegan diet before.

When you are ready to see some major changes in your health from weight loss to increased energy make sure to check out this guidebook to get the tools, and recipes that you need, to begin.

Thank you again for purchasing this book!

I hope this book was able to help introduce you to the Vegan diet and provide Vegan recipes for you to enjoy.

The next step is to immediately convert to Veganism, COMMIT to it and REAP the rewards!

Finally, if you enjoyed this book, then I'd like to ask you for a favor, would you be kind enough to leave a review for this book on Amazon? It'd be greatly appreciated!

Thank you and good luck!

43303048R00029

Made in the USA
Middletown, DE
06 May 2017